FERTILITY DIET, THE INFERTILITY KILLER

NATURAL WAYS TO IMPROVE FERTILITY EVEN @40'S

CLARE DOMINIC

ISBN: 9798849468686

Imprint: Independently published

Cover design by: Art Painter

Library of Congress Control Number: 20195375309

Printed in the United States of America

DEDICATION

This book is dedicated to all spouses having difficulty in conception. Don't be emotional because your worries will be over soon. You will carry your Baby sooner than you expected.

Just do the needful and develop a positive mindset. Success!!

Author's Note

Dear Reader,

Thank you for picking up this book. Whether you are just starting your fertility journey or have been on this path for some time, I want you to know this: you are not alone, and you are already taking an incredible step forward by seeking knowledge and support.

I wrote this guide to help women (and couples) understand the powerful connection between nutrition and fertility. My goal is to offer you simple, science— backed advice that can make a meaningful difference —no hype, no empty promises, just practical tools you can use right away.

Remember, this journey is not just about getting to a positive pregnancy test — it's also about strengthening your body, balancing your health, and creating the best foundation for the little one you're hoping to welcome.

With hope and encouragement,

Clare Dominic

Table of Contents

INTRODUCTION

What you put on your plate can play a powerful role in helping you conceive the baby you've been dreaming of.

In this guide, you'll discover the most beneficial foods and nutrients that can naturally increase your chances of getting pregnant — whether you're in your 20s, 30s, or even your 40s.

We've long known that nutrition shapes our overall health, but what many couples don't realize is just how deeply food choices can influence fertility.

Certain foods have been shown to improve the quality of ovulation in women, enhance sperm health in men, and create the ideal conditions for conception. But the big question remains: **what exactly should you put on your plate to boost your fertility and maximize your chances of success?**

This book will guide you step by step through the essential foods, vitamins, minerals, and lifestyle strategies that can help you nourish your body, balance your hormones, and prepare for the journey to parenthood.

CHAPTER ONE

Foods That Can Boost Your Fertility

Getting pregnant, some happen in the blink of an eye, others have to put in a little more effort to boost fertility. Whichever group you fall into, it is always wise to adjust your diet.

For example, it is a good idea to avoid soda, fast food and other unhealthy products. But did you know that there are also foods that can have a positive effect on your fertility?

10x Foods That Promote Fertility

Here are ten foods you can eat more often if you're trying to conceive:

Seeds

Seeds such as linseed, chia seed and hemp seed can contribute to better fertility because of the omega 3 fatty acids they contain. Several studies have established that omega 3 can increase the fertility of both men and women. Add the seeds as a topping to a salad, smoothie, oatmeal or yogurt.

Poultry

If you want to get pregnant, it's a good idea to put chicken or turkey on the menu more often. Poultry can support the fertility of women. It can also improve sperm quality in men.

sunflower seeds

Sunflower seeds are rich in folic acid, which makes them an excellent food for anyone who wants to have children. The B vitamin is not only important for the healthy development of the unborn child, but also has a positive effect on fertility.

Sprinkle sunflower seeds over salads or try sunflower seed butter on a healthy cracker of nuts, seeds and kernels.

Fatty fish

Fatty fish contains various nutrients with a positive effect on fertility. To be precise: omega—3 fatty acids, vitamin B12 and vitamin D. Especially omega—3 fatty acids can have a positive effect on the fertility of women.

Vitamin D can help improve menstrual frequency and improve sperm quality. To take full advantage of the beneficial effect of oily fish, it is best to choose fish with the least mercury. Think of sardines, mackerel, herring, trout and salmon.

walnuts

Walnuts are not only good for your brain, but also for your fertility. They contain quite a lot of omega 3 fatty acids.

Whole grains

Whole grains can promote fertility in women and improve sperm quality in men. However, grains such as wheat and spelled also contain a lot of carbohydrates. Therefore, they are not such a good idea if you are overweight and want to lose weight to increase the chance of pregnancy.

Oatmeal is a good alternative if you want to get pregnant and lose weight healthily. This cereal contains carbohydrates that are good for you.

pistachios

Do you like pistachios? They are great if you want to get pregnant, because they contain quite a lot of omega 3, which supports fertility.

Vegetables fruit

Fruits and vegetables are always a good idea, especially if you want to increase your fertility. There is a clear link between these natural products and better fertility in women. In men, semen quality is said to improve by eating fruits and vegetables.

Green leafy vegetables in particular are high in folic acid, which is known to promote fertility. A fruit like pineapple provides many antioxidants that can improve sperm quality in men undergoing fertility treatment.

Soy

Soy is rich in folic acid, which is beneficial if you want to get pregnant. The legume appears to have a particularly beneficial effect on the fertility of women undergoing fertility treatment.

Seafood

Research shows that couples who eat more seafood are more likely to get pregnant than people who rarely have seafood on the menu. Mussels in particular are rich in vitamin B12, which has a beneficial effect on the fertility of both women and men. All the more reason to include these and other seafood in your diet.

Eat yourself pregnant! 6x nutrition tips to increase your fertility

Scenario one: you want to have children. You discuss this with your partner and together you think it is time for a family expansion. You stop contraception, buy a new lingerie set and spend the necessary hours under the sheets. A month later you buy a test et voila: you look enthusiastically at two red stripes. Very nice if this goes so smoothly, but this scenario is often the exception to the rule. Do you want to contribute to increasing your fertility yourself? Then your eating habits can influence that.

Research shows that (among other things) your diet and BMI can influence your fertility. Of course, there are many factors involved in a successful pregnancy. In any case, you want to make sure that it can't be your diet.

Increase your fertility

The next time you're standing in front of the fridge, think about this list before you go for the wine bottle. These nutritional tips can help you increase your fertility.

1. Eat Antioxidants

Whether a family expansion is planned or not, eating enough fruits and vegetables can of course never hurt. Especially if you want to increase your fertility, it is important to get enough antioxidants. You have to deal with all kinds of free radicals in your body on a daily basis. Sounds nasty , but this is completely normal. If you get enough antioxidants, that's not a problem at all. So eat plenty of fruits and vegetables, nuts and seeds: these are packed with antioxidants such as vitamins C and E. Also for the guys by the way! So nice to crack walnuts together!

2. Big breakfast

Especially if you suffer from PCOS, it is wise to start with a large breakfast. With PCOS there is a problem with your insulin , and this balance can be restored if you start the morning with a big breakfast.

3. Eat Other Carbs

We now have a love/hate relationship with carbohydrates. We all know that we should not eat too much of it, but the type of carbohydrates can also affect your fertility. Especially avoid the refined carbohydrates. These have a high glycemic index (GI) , an index that can determine how much sugar is in food, which in turn determines your insulin. So it is useful to know which ingredients are high and low in GI. The bottom line: fruits and vegetables are low. Bread, pasta, rice are high.

Eat More Fiber

Fiber is not only good for your gut, but also for your hormone balance. The hormone estrogen is broken down in your liver, enters our intestines and then leaves our body through urine and feces. So make sure you get enough (but not too much) fiber. It is recommended to eat between 30 and 40 grams of fiber per day. Oops, we can improve on that: on average, the Dutch eat between 15 and 23 grams per day.

5. Cut Down Your Caffeine

Ai, bad news for the coffee addicts among us. KarlijnHoebe , nutritionist specialized in hormone balance, therefore recommends drinking (and eating) less caffeine if you want to increase your fertility. You find caffeine not only in coffee and some teas, but also in chocolate and cola.

6. Check your iron intake

Is your iron intake too low? Then you can feel tired, and

have a pale face. You can then increase your iron by eating iron— rich foods, or opt for an iron supplement. Still, there are mixed feelings about taking iron supplements, as too high an iron level can have a negative effect on your fertility. So check it out with your doctor if you want to increase your fertility.

If you stick to all the nutrition tips, and have the feeling that something else is going on, then don't doubt yourself. Many factors can play a role, so be sure to check with your doctor. The sooner you rule out other factors, the sooner you know what's going on.

Do you want children but not yet pregnant? Try a fertility massage!

Suppose you want to have children, but you have not been able to get pregnant until now. That can be very frustrating. A fertility massage could help you with this!

What exactly is a fertility massage, where can you have it done and how can it speed up the process of getting pregnant? We explain it in this article.

What is a fertility massage?

A fertility massage is a massage of your abdomen and lower back. The way you are massaged is aimed at increasing blood flow to your reproductive organs. That's your ovaries and uterus.

Normally, only 3% of all your blood supply flows through your uterus and ovaries. While research shows that if these organs get more blood flow, they can do their job better.

The quality of your eggs will improve and massage will put less stress on your uterus. This allows the lining of the womb to build up better, increasing your chances of pregnancy.

You will also notice that your periods become less painful. This is because much of the tension built up in this area is removed by the massage.

Who is a fertility massage suitable for?

In principle, a fertility massage is suitable for anyone who has a wish to have children, but has not yet seen it come true:

Women who want to get pregnant, but have not succeeded so far

Massage is also suitable for women who have experienced a miscarriage or stillbirth

Women who are in an IVF or ICSI process

As soon as you lose confidence in your body, massage is also very suitable for you

Women who want to experience fewer complaints during their menstrual period

The best time to book a massage

The most ideal time to book a fertility massage is in the period between your period and ovulation. It is wise not to book a massage during your period.

During the first intake you will be asked many questions. About your own health, your work, your relationship and of course your wish to have children. By gathering this information, the therapists can create a treatment plan that is right for you.

CHAPTER TWO

Let's Talk About Fertility, Hope, and the Vitamins That Really Matter

You know, when my best friend Lily and her husband started trying for a baby, they thought it'd happen like clockwork. She ditched the pill, they high— fived each other, and figured they'd be shopping for onesies by the end of the year. Fast forward 14 months, and she was knee -- deep in ovulation tests and sobbing quietly during baby food commercials. It was brutal.

That's when we started digging into the stuff no one really talks about — like how your body needs *actual nutrients*, not just hope and a calendar app, to get the baby ball rolling. Turns out, vitamins and minerals aren't just good for your skin or nails — they're *foundational* for healthy eggs and strong swimmers.

Real Talk: What's Actually Going on In There?

Eggs and sperm aren't made overnight. It takes *months* for them to mature, and during that time, your body's working behind the scenes, doing the delicate work of DNA replication, hormone balancing, and cellular repair. It's like tending a garden — if the soil's not rich, nothing's going to **grow right.**

That's where these key players come in…

Folate (aka folic acid, but better in methylated form)

When Lily's doctor finally brought up folate, she sighed and said, "Isn't that just for pregnant women?" Nope. Not even close. Folate is critical for egg development and for sperm to form properly. It's like giving your DNA a protective bubble wrap. And guys need it too —it helps reduce chromosomal abnormalities.

Lily switched to a prenatal with methylfolate (the bioavailable kind) and *swears* it made her cycles feel more predictable. "It was like my body finally exhaled," she told me.

Zinc: The Unsung Hero

Let me tell you about Joe, my coworker. Super healthy guy, gym every morning, no major vices. But his sperm count? Tanked. His doc took one look at his diet and said, "Dude, you need more zinc." Turns out, zinc is vital for testosterone production and sperm motility — you know, the ability of those little guys to swim like Olympic athletes. He started eating more pumpkin seeds and shellfish (hello oysters!) and taking a quality supplement. Six months later, they were staring at a positive test.

CoQ10: Like Coffee for Your Cells

Lily's RE (reproductive endocrinologist) suggested this one — not cheap, but worth it. CoQ10 gives your cells the energy they need, especially the mitochondria in your eggs. It's like rocket fuel for egg quality, especially if you're in your 30s or 40s and feeling the pressure of the "biological clock."

She said it was like her body "woke up." Her energy went up, and emotionally, she felt more *in control*. Fertility treatments can make you feel like a passenger in your own life — anything that gives you back some agency? That's gold.

Vitamin D: Not Just for Bones

This one hit close to home. I live in a cloudy part of the country, and my own vitamin D levels were always in the gutter. When I was trying to conceive, my OB tested me and was like, "Well no wonder your hormones are all over the place." Vitamin D acts like a hormone itself —it influences ovarian reserve, hormone balance, and sperm development.

I now call my morning walk my "fertility walk." A little sunshine, a little grounding, a moment to breathe.

Omega—3s: The Lube for Your Reproductive System

Okay, not literally. But omega—3 fatty acids reduce inflammation and improve blood flow to the ovaries and testes. That means better egg maturation and improved sperm shape and function. A friend of mine with PCOS (who always had weird cycles) said after she started taking fish oil, her cycles became more regular. She laughed, "I think my ovaries finally chilled out."

Magnesium, Iron, and B12: The Support Crew

These three don't always get the spotlight, but trust me, they're working overtime behind the scenes. Magnesium helps with hormone regulation and stress (because stress is *hell* on fertility). Iron is essential for healthy ovulation, and B12 helps both egg and sperm quality— especially important if you're vegan or vegetarian.

The Emotional Side of All This

Can I just say something here? This journey is not just about test results and supplements. It's about heartbreak, and hope, and quiet perseverance. It's about checking your app every morning, wondering if this will be *the month*. It's about eating Brazil nuts because someone on a Facebook group swore by it, and crying in the grocery store because a kid asked their mom if she had a baby in her belly.

So yeah — vitamins help. A lot. But *you* matter more. Your hope, your heart, your grit.

If you're navigating this path right now, please know you're not alone. There are little things you can do that make a big difference —in your body, your mindset, and your future family.

And if you ever need someone to say, "You're doing enough," let that be me. You are. You really are.

xxix

CHAPTER THREE

Where Do I Even Start?" – The Basics on a Budget

If you're just beginning your fertility journey and don't want to drop $$$ on supplements right away, start with this **core trio** — solid for both egg and sperm health:

- **Prenatal with methylfolate**: Don't skimp on this. Get one with *methylfolate, not* synthetic folic acid (especially if you have the MTHFR gene mutation — more common than you'd think). I like Thorne or MegaFood, but even some store brands now offer the methyl version.

- **Vitamin D3 (2,000–4,000 IU daily)**: If you don't get much sun, this is a nonnegotiable. I take it with breakfast and no drama.

- **Omega—3 (DHA + EPA)**: Look for one that doesn't taste like fish burps, trust me. Nordic Naturals is great, and Costco even has a decent option.

FREE *TIP:* Buy in bulk online, and consider a daily pill organizer. It saves sanity *and* dollars.

I Have PCOS and My Hormones Are All Over the Place

You're not imagining it — PCOS can be a rollercoaster. But it's not a dead end. I've seen real magic happen with targeted support.

- **Inositol (myo + d—chiro blend, ideally 40:1 ratio)**: Total game— changer. Helps with insulin sensitivity, regulates cycles, and supports egg quality. Ovasitol is a fan favorite — tastes like nothing and dissolves in water.

- **Magnesium glycinate**: For stress, sleep, and smoother hormones. Most women are low in magnesium anyway.

- **Omega—3s**: PCOS often means chronic inflammation, and this helps cool the fire.

- **Zinc + Vitamin D**: Helps with androgen levels (acne, hair growth, etc.) and ovulation support.

My cousin Sarah had cycles like, once every four months. After 3 months of inositol + magnesium, her period came back on the dot. Her OB was like, "Okay, what are you doing differently?" She said, "I started treating my body like it deserved rhythm, not chaos."

"I'm 35+ and Feeling the Pressure"

Whew, the "advanced maternal age" label stings, doesn't it? But listen- your eggs are *not* doomed. You've got tools.

- **CoQ10 (Ubiquinol form, 200–400mg/day)**: This is the holy grail for mitochondrial health in eggs and sperm. Don't skimp here.

- **Vitamin E + C**: They're antioxidants that protect fragile egg cells from oxidative stress — especially important over 35.

- **Prenatal with *methylated* B vitamins**: B12, folate, B6, all matter more as we age.

- **NAC (N—acetylcysteine)**: Especially if you're going through IVF —it helps with egg maturation and can improve egg retrieval quality.

My friend Rachel started these at 39. She was told she'd need donor eggs —6 months later, she had two viable embryos from her own retrieval. "I just wanted one more chance," she said. And she got it.

"My Partner's Sperm Test Came Back... Not Great"

Men get sidelined in fertility convos *way* too often. But sperm health is half the equation and there's *a lot* they can do.

- **Zinc (25–40mg/day)**: Improves count and motility. Also boosts testosterone levels naturally.

- **Vitamin C & E**: Antioxidants protect sperm from DNA damage.

- **CoQ10 (200–300mg/day)**: Sperm are *very* energy, hungry. This helps them swim like they mean it.

- **L—Carnitine & L—Arginine**: Improve motility and morphology — the shape and movement of sperm.

- **Ashwagandha or Maca** (optional, depending on stress/testosterone): Can help with libido, stress, and sperm concentration. Just get a high—quality one — not gas station nonsense.

Real guy story: Mike, a buddy from college, hated the idea of taking "fertility supplements." But after three months on CoQ10 and a zinc blend, his motility went from 28% to 64%. His wife? Pregnant on the next cycle. He now calls it his "super sperm stack."

"I'm Going Through IVF – Help Me Maximize My Chances"

You're brave. I see you. IVF can feel like a medical boot camp, but supplements can truly support the process.

- **CoQ10 (again!)**: Yes, this again. It supports embryo quality and egg development. Essential.

- **Vitamin D + Omega—3**: Helps with implantation, inflammation, and mood —all important for IVF success.

- **Melatonin (low dose, like 2–3mg at night)**: Weirdly, yes - melatonin has been shown to support egg maturation and follicle quality during IVF cycles.

- **NAC + Alpha Lipoic Acid (ALA)**: Both support egg retrieval and embryo development by fighting oxidative stress.

- **Prenatal + B—complex**: Keeps your baseline nutrients strong while your body is doing all. the. things.

Pro hack: Start your stack 2–3 months before stimulation — egg quality is set well before retrieval day.

Please NOTE: This whole journey? It's part science, part heart, and part stubborn hope. Supplements are *tools*, not magic pills. They don't replace sleep, nourishing food, or real emotional care — but they sure as hell can tip the scales in your favor.

And you deserve to feel like you're doing *something*. Something powerful. Something that says, "Hey, I haven't given up."

I've got your back. If you want a personalized regimen or

want help reading your labs or supplement labels, I'm happy

to walk through it with you. Just say the word.

CHAPTER FOUR

How to Improve Ovulation and Hormone Balance
Naturally

**Am I Even Ovulating?" Now Let's Talk About
Hormones, Hope, and Healing Naturally**

When you're trying to get pregnant and your body isn't
playing along, it's easy to start feeling like a stranger inside
your own skin. I've been there. And so have a dozen of my
closest friends —whispering to each other about
temperatures and cervical mucus and that weird pain near the
left ovary that maybe means something... or maybe just
means tacos.

So many of us never really learn how ovulation *actually* works
until it's not working right. And then it hits like a freight train:
the 45—day cycles, the "your progesterone is low" lab calls,
the crushed hope at yet another negative test.

But I want you to know —there are ways to nudge your body
back into rhythm. Gentle, natural ways. No miracle cures

here, just honest—to—goodness support for a system that's probably more tired than broken.

Finding Your Flow Again (Literally)

Take Emily, for example. She hadn't had a period in six months —not since coming off birth control. She thought they'd just snap back. Instead, she found herself stuck in a hormonal limbo: always waiting, always googling, always second—guessing.

Her doctor told her to "just wait." But waiting felt like standing still. So, she started small —really small.

"I started eating breakfast again," she told me one night, laughing through tears. "Like, *real* breakfast. Protein, fat, carbs. Not just coffee and vibes."

That tiny change? It was a game—changer. Turns out, your hormones *need* blood sugar stability. Your ovaries are picky —

they don't ovulate when they think you're starving, stressed, or skipping meals.

Two months of consistent eating, and boom —her period returned. Three cycles later, she ovulated on day 16. The kind of win that feels bigger than a win.

Eat Like You Love Your Hormones

I'm not going to tell you to "just go keto" or cut out every carb. Honestly, that kind of stuff messed me up more than it helped. What helped me (and a lot of others)?

Real food. Balanced meals. Less noise.

Things like:

- Eggs with the yolk. Don't fear fat —your hormones *need* cholesterol.

- Leafy greens. Think spinach, arugula, chard —full of magnesium and folate.

- Sweet potatoes. Especially if you have PCOS or irregular cycles. They're grounding.

- Seeds —like pumpkin and flax in the first half of your cycle, sesame and sunflower in the second (aka **seed cycling** —kind of woo, kind of wonderful).

- Bone broth. I know it sounds weird, but for folks with thin uterine lining or wonky cycles? It's rich in collagen, minerals, and warmth. Feels like a hug from the inside.

The Stress Hormone Nobody Talks About Enough

Can we talk about cortisol? The big bad wolf of hormone balance?

Because honestly, it's the most overlooked piece of this puzzle.

When you're chronically stressed (and let's be real —fertility struggles are *stress embodied*), your body redirects its energy toward survival, not reproduction. It's not personal. It's just biology. But it *feels* personal, doesn't it?

Nora, a yoga teacher I met at a hormone retreat, told me how she got her ovulation back by *slowing down*. Not quitting her life. Just... softening her mornings. Meditating 10 minutes. Walking instead of jogging. Saying no without guilt. And maybe most importantly, sleeping before midnight.

Three months of being kind to her nervous system, and her LH surge (aka the sign of ovulation) came back. "I thought I needed more supplements," she said. "I just needed less **chaos.**"

Herbs That Whisper to Your Hormones

I'm not a doctor, but I've had tea with enough herbalists to tell you —plants can help.

- **Vitex (chasteberry)**: Good for low progesterone, irregular cycles, or after coming off birth control. But not great if you have PCOS or high LH —so ask around.

- **Maca root**: A Peruvian root that helps with energy and libido. Some women *swear* by it for balancing estrogen and progesterone.

- **Spearmint tea**: For those with PCOS and high androgens (think chin hair, acne, oily skin) —it can reduce testosterone naturally.

- **Ashwagandha**: A gentle adaptogen. Helps your adrenals chill out so your ovaries can come back online.

I always say: herbs don't "fix" you —they *support* you. Like little green allies in your journey.

Ovulation Is a Love Letter From Your Body

It's your body's way of saying: "I'm nourished. I'm rested. I feel safe."

So if it's not happening right now? That doesn't mean you're broken. It might just mean your body needs time, or support, or a new kind of kindness.

My own cycle disappeared after a bad breakup and a year of overworking myself. I was running on caffeine and adrenaline, sleeping four hours a night, trying to be "fine." When I finally let myself fall apart —and then rebuilt my life on softer ground —my cycle came back. And with it, my sense of self.

You're Not Alone in This

If you're reading this and your heart's aching, I see you.

Whether you're 22 or 42, whether you're trying to conceive or just want your cycle to *make sense* again —know this: your body wants to work with you. It's not fighting you. It's just asking for help in its own quiet language.

Listen gently.

Eat the damn yolk. Take the walk. Say no to things that drain you. Say yes to joy, even in small stolen moments.

Ovulation isn't just a physical process —it's a sign of vitality, rhythm, and life moving through you.

And I believe in your body's ability to come back to balance —naturally, and in its own time.

CHAPTER FIVE

Top Foods for Hormone Balance (And How to Eat Them Without Getting Bored)

When you're trying to get your hormones to chill out and work *with* you instead of against you, what you eat matters more than we've been taught to believe. Not in a fear—based, restriction—heavy kind of way. But in a nourishing, supportive, "Hey body, I got you" kind of way.

These five ingredients are legit rockstars for hormone harmony:

Leafy greens

Think spinach, kale, arugula, chard. These babies are rich in **folate and magnesium**, which help regulate your cycle, support egg health, and calm the nervous system.

Eggs

A whole—food, fertility—friendly staple. Eggs are loaded with **protein, choline** (which supports fetal brain development), and **vitamin D,** which helps regulate ovulation.

Berries

They're not just cute and sweet —they're **packed with antioxidants** that fight off inflammation and protect those precious reproductive cells.

Brazil nuts

Even just *1–2 a day* can supply you with your daily **selenium,** a mineral that protects the thyroid and supports progesterone production.

Maca root

An ancient **adaptogen** that supports hormone balance, energy, and libido. Best used in powder form —think smoothies, oatmeal, or energy bites

7—Day Meal Plan for Happy Hormones (That Tastes Like Real Life)

Here's a week of hormone hugging meals you'll actually *want* to eat. Nothing fancy, no guilt trips, just real food that feels good in your body.

Day 1

Breakfast:

Scrambled eggs with spinach and avocado on sourdough toast
Cook in a little olive oil, toss in some baby spinach, season with salt and pepper. Top with sliced avo and chili flakes.

Lunch:

Quinoa salad with kale, roasted sweet potato, chickpeas, and tahini dressing

Toss everything together and drizzle with lemon—tahini sauce.

Dinner:

Baked salmon with garlic sautéed chard and wild rice
Squeeze fresh lemon over the fish, add a few crushed Brazil nuts on top for crunch.

Snack:

Handful of blueberries + 2 Brazil nuts

Day 2

Breakfast:

Maca berry smoothie (almond milk, frozen blueberries, banana, flaxseeds, 1 tsp maca)
Blend until creamy. Optional scoop of collagen or plant protein.

Lunch:

Turkey lettuce wraps with cucumber, hummus, and shredded carrots
Wrap it all in big romaine leaves. Super refreshing and low—glycemic.

Dinner:

Zucchini noodles with ground turkey, spinach, and tomato basil sauce
Quick sauté with garlic and onions. Sprinkle with nutritional yeast or parm.

Snack:

Hard—boiled egg + a few strawberries

Day 3

Breakfast:

Oatmeal with ground flaxseed, cinnamon, blueberries, and a drizzle of almond butter
Add maca powder to the mix if you're into it.

Lunch:

Spinach and goat cheese frittata + arugula side salad with lemon vinaigrette
Make a big batch —it reheats beautifully.

Dinner:

Chicken stir—fry with kale, broccoli, and sesame oil over brown rice
Use coconut aminos instead of soy sauce for a hormone—friendly twist.

Snack:

Dark chocolate square + 1 Brazil nut

Day 4

Breakfast:

Greek yogurt bowl with berries, pumpkin seeds, and a dash of maca
Try full—fat if you tolerate dairy well —the fat helps with hormone production.

Lunch:

Lentil soup with kale and turmeric + a slice of whole grain bread
Warming and grounding —add lemon for brightness.

Dinner:

Stuffed bell peppers with quinoa, ground beef, spinach, and chopped Brazil nuts
Roast until soft and golden. So satisfying.

Snack:

Apple slices with almond butter

Day 5

Breakfast:

Egg muffins with chopped greens, mushrooms, and goat cheese
Bake in muffin tins for grab—and—go ease.

Lunch:

Tuna salad with olive oil mayo, arugula, and avocado on seed crackers
Add pickles if you're feeling spicy.

Dinner:

Coconut curry with tofu, kale, and brown rice
Toss in some sweet potatoes and finish with cilantro.
Comfort in a bowl.

Snack:

Mixed berries and a handful of walnuts

Day 6

Breakfast:

Smoothie bowl with frozen berries, spinach, chia seeds, maca, and granola

So pretty. So good.

Lunch:

Chopped kale salad with eggs, avocado, sunflower seeds, and tahini—lemon dressing
Massage the kale to make it tender and delicious.

Dinner:

Grilled chicken with roasted Brussels sprouts and garlic mashed sweet potatoes
Add rosemary or thyme for cozy, earthy flavor.

Snack:

Coconut yogurt with cinnamon + 1 Brazil nut

Day 7

Breakfast:

Avocado toast topped with poached egg and arugula
Sprinkle of hemp seeds for extra hormone love.

Lunch:

Buddha bowl with quinoa, chickpeas, roasted veggies, and tahini dressing
A catch—all for leftovers —nourishing and colorful.

Dinner:

Maca mushroom risotto with sautéed greens Cook slowly with broth and finish with a splash of coconut milk. Fancy—feeling but totally weeknight—friendly.

Snack:

Berry smoothie + a square of dark chocolate

It's important to note that Food can be so healing. Not just because of what's *in* it —the nutrients, the macros, the superfoods —but because of how it makes you *feel*. Empowered. Cared for. Connected.

Don't worry about being perfect. If you make scrambled eggs and toss some greens on the side, that's a hormone win. If you snack on berries instead of chips one afternoon? That's a win. If you drink water before your third coffee? Huge win.

Your body is listening. And it wants to feel better, just like you do.

CHAPTER SIX

The Fertility Diet Mistakes Most Couples Make (and How to Gently Fix Them)

I remember sitting at a coffee shop with my friend Lila, both of us nursing overpriced oat milk lattes and a mountain of quiet frustration. She had just said, "I'm eating *so clean*… like, quinoa and kale and no sugar, not even fruit. So why the hell aren't we pregnant yet?"

She wasn't looking for a nutritional breakdown. She was looking for *relief*. And honestly? That moment hit me like a ton of bricks. Because I'd done the same thing micromanaging every bite, obsessively reading food blogs at 2 a.m., cutting out everything but still feeling like I was doing it all wrong.

Turns out, a lot of us are making the same food mistakes

when we're trying to conceive and we don't even know it.

Let's talk about some of them. Honestly. Lovingly. With a side of grace.

Mistake #1: "Clean Eating" That's *Too* Clean

There's this thing that happens when you start googling "fertility foods." Suddenly, your knee deep in diet culture dressed up as wellness. Everything's about elimination: no dairy, no gluten, no sugar, no caffeine, no joy, no flavor.

I had a client once —let's call her Jess —who was eating grilled chicken, steamed broccoli, and brown rice on repeat. No sauces. No oils. No snacks unless they were "approved." She was exhausted. Her cycle was all over the place. Her libido? Gone. Her relationship? On edge.

The fix? We *added* food back in. Full—fat yogurt with berries. A couple of eggs each morning. Dark chocolate at night.

Butter, for God's sake. She emailed me two months later: "I got my period on time for the first time in a year. Also, I'm actually enjoying food again."

Eating *clean* doesn't mean eating *empty*. Fertility thrives on nourishment, not deprivation.

Mistake #2: Forgetting That Men Eat Too

Can we normalize talking about *his* diet too?

Because I swear, every couple I talk to starts with, "I've cut caffeine and added maca and I'm taking three different prenatals," and then adds, "He's...uh...trying to eat more nuts?"

It's not a blame game. It's biology. Sperm are just as vulnerable to oxidative stress, nutrient deficiencies, and inflammation. A guy's diet affects motility, morphology, count —all of it. But nobody really tells them that.

I had a friend whose husband was drinking two energy drinks a day, skipping meals, and living on takeout. She was doing acupuncture and tracking basal temps. He didn't even know what a folate supplement was.

The shift came when they started cooking together. Making dinner became a "we" thing —salmon with roasted sweet potatoes, green smoothies in the morning, weekend meal prep. Less pressure, more partnership. She said, "It finally felt like we were in this together."

Mistake #3: Getting Obsessed with "Fertility Superfoods"

Listen. I *love* a good fertility superfood moment. Give me maca root, bee pollen, spirulina, goji berries, flaxseeds —I've bought them all. But here's the thing: you can sprinkle chia seeds on a donut and it's still a donut.

What actually matters? **Consistency**. Not perfection. Not

spending $400 on adaptogens. Not eating goji berries flown in from the mountains of Tibet.

When you zoom out, fertility nutrition isn't about finding magic foods —it's about stabilizing blood sugar, calming inflammation, supporting gut health, and making sure your hormones feel safe enough to do their thing.

And honestly? Half of that can be done with regular—ass food. Eggs. Greens. Avocados. Whole grains. Water. Real meals. That's it. No wizardry required.

Mistake #4: Skipping Meals (Especially Breakfast)

If I had a dollar for every woman who told me, "I just don't feel hungry in the morning," I'd have... a lot of dollars and a room full of dysregulated hormones.

Skipping breakfast messes with your blood sugar and cortisol, which —surprise! —messes with ovulation. Your body sees it as stress. And stress tells your body, "Now is not the time to reproduce."

I used to think fasting until noon was "clean" and "disciplined." But my period didn't agree. When I started eating breakfast —something warm, with fat and protein — my cycle got shorter and less chaotic.

Try scrambled eggs on toast. Or oatmeal with almond butter. Or a smoothie with spinach, chia, and banana. You don't have to be fancy. You just have to *feed yourself.*

Mistake #5: Doing It All Alone

This one's sneaky. Because technically, it's not a diet mistake. But it *shows up* in how we eat —in isolation, in shame, in secrecy.

So many women are quietly cutting food groups, hiding supplements in their purse, crying over pasta. Feeling guilty for having a glass of wine at dinner. Skipping brunch because it doesn't "fit the plan."

Fertility can be a lonely road. But it doesn't have to be.

My best meals were the ones I shared —with friends who didn't judge, with my partner when we cooked messy pasta together, with my sister over a shared chocolate bar. That connection *is* nourishment too. And you need both.

So How Do We Fix It?

Honestly? You just start where you are. With what you have.

You feed yourself enough. You stop trying to be a perfect food robot. You share the journey with your partner. You eat carbs (yes, carbs). You remember that this isn't a punishment. It's preparation.

Fertility isn't just about getting pregnant —it's about creating a body that feels safe, nourished, and whole. That kind of body is ready for life —in every sense of the word.

And if you ever forget that, come back to this one small truth: **your body wants to work with you**. It just needs a little help —and maybe a slice of sourdough.

CHAPTER SEVEN

A Simple Meal Plan to Support Your Baby Journey

(For real people, with real cravings, and real busy lives)

There's a moment I'll never forget. I was sitting on the kitchen floor, back against the fridge, eating a spoonful of peanut butter straight from the jar. I had just gotten my period again —late, painful, discouraging. I remember thinking, "I'm doing everything right. The supplements. The charting. The eating clean. What more does my body want?"

And that's when something clicked.

This journey? It's not just about the baby. It's about coming back to *yourself*. Taking care of your body in a way that's about love —not control.

So this meal plan? It's built on that. Simple food. Warm, grounding meals. A little indulgence. A lot of nourishment. No stress.

Morning Vibes – Gentle Starts That Feed Your Hormones

Real talk: Your hormones are *begging* for a good breakfast. Skipping meals might feel productive, but it's one of the fastest ways to mess with ovulation. Your body wants to feel safe —and fed.

Sample Morning:

- **Warm oatmeal with ground flaxseed, chia, almond butter, and berries**
  This was my go—to. I'd stir it all together in a pot with almond milk and a pinch of cinnamon. The fats and fiber kept me full, and flax is amazing for estrogen balance.
- **Or try:**

o   Scrambled eggs with spinach and avocado

o   A smoothie with banana, spinach, collagen, and a spoon of peanut butter

I had a client, Sarah, who swore she "wasn't a breakfast person." But we started small —a slice of sprouted toast with nut butter. Within a few weeks, her blood sugar steadied, her mood lifted, and her cycles became more regular. "Turns out," she told me, "my body *does* like breakfast —just not at 7 a.m."

Midday Meals – Energy Without the Slump

Lunch should be filling, grounding, and easy to prep ahead (especially if you're juggling work, appointments, or just... life). You're not trying to impress anyone here. You're feeding future follicles. That's sacred.

Sample Lunch:

- **Quinoa bowl with roasted veggies, chickpeas, kale, and tahini lemon dressing**

  I batch this on Sundays. Roasted sweet potatoes, zucchini, bell peppers —whatever's on hand. Add some protein (like lentils or salmon) and greens, drizzle with tahini. Boom.

- **Other faves:**

  o Chicken salad with avocado, mixed greens, and olive oil

  o Lentil soup with spinach and a slice of sourdough

  o Tuna on rye with arugula and pickles (underrated and SO good)

One couple I worked with made lunch their "daily fertility check—in." They'd prep together, sit down at the table (even for just 20 minutes), and talk about how they were feeling —

not just physically, but emotionally. It became their ritual. She said it saved their relationship during the rough patches.

Evening Eats – Calm, Cozy, and Hormone—Friendly

Dinner doesn't need to be gourmet. But try to make it warm, rich in protein and good fats, and ideally something you look forward to —not just something you toss together on autopilot.

Sample Dinner:

- **Grilled salmon with garlicky sautéed kale and roasted baby potatoes** Omega—3s from the salmon, magnesium from the kale, comforting carbs from the potatoes. A hormone hug on a plate.

- **Other comfort combos:**
  - Stir—fried tofu with broccoli, carrots, and brown rice

- o Grass—fed beef chili with beans and a slice of cornbread

- o Pasta with pesto, peas, and poached egg on top (trust me —it slaps)

I remember cooking this chickpea curry one night after a tough appointment. My partner and I were quiet the whole time. But as we sat down to eat, something softened. "This feels like hope," he said. Sometimes, dinner is more than just food. It's healing.

Snacks and Sweets – Yes, You *Can* Have Dessert

Don't let anyone convince you that enjoying food is somehow bad for fertility. If dark chocolate and dates dipped in peanut butter are wrong, I don't want to be right.

- **Snack ideas:**

- o A boiled egg with hummus

- o Brazil nuts (just 1–2 a day for selenium!)

- o   Greek yogurt with berries and cinnamon

- o   Sliced apple with tahini drizzle

- **Sweet treats that love you back:**

    - o   A square (or two) of dark chocolate

    - o   Chia pudding with coconut milk and mango

    - o   Baked pear with cinnamon and almond butter

Take this…. (From Someone Who's Been There)

If you take anything from this, let it be this: **your body is not broken**. It's doing everything it can to protect you, to keep you steady, to prepare.

The baby journey can feel long. Some days you'll feel powerful. Some days you'll cry into your soup. All of it is valid.

But when you feed yourself —truly nourish yourself —you're telling your body: *I trust you. I believe in you. I love you even before you give me what I want.*

That's powerful.

CHAPTER EIGHT

Could a cold uterus be the reason you are not getting pregnant?

A cold uterus. I had never heard of it. Cold Uterus is a concept in Chinese medicine that means that the uterus (or rather the mucous membrane) does not respond well to the hormone progesterone that helps an embryo to implant. Result: it is difficult to get pregnant. How do you know if this is bothering you? And most importantly, what can you do about it?

How do you recognize a cold uterus?

Women who suffer from a cold uterus can be recognized by a basal body temperature rising too slowly or falling too quickly. Characteristics that can indicate cold hands and feet, a somewhat darker and thicker menstrual period, lower back pain, a low libido (less sex drive) and frequent urination at night.

Like a seed in the ground that won't pop up in cold weather, it's harder for an embryo to nest and grow if the temperature of its habitat is 'too cold'. This view of a woman's womb comes from natural medicine.

At conception between a sperm cell and egg cell to embryo, the implantation time is approximately one week. A uterus that is in a sub—optimal condition cannot always provide the embryo with the right environment to become pregnant. With possible miscarriage as a result.

According to alternative medicine, eating raw foods, drinking cold drinks, cold weather and cold environments, being a vegetarian and eating too much cold energy foods such as raw fruits and vegetables has a (negative) influence on the uterus.

Solution for a cold uterus

The treatment plan for a woman with this condition is to warm the uterus so that the progesterone functions optimally in the body. The uterus can then work optimally because it provides the best possible nourishing environment.

In alternative and Chinese medicine, acupuncture and herbal therapies are said to help improve blood circulation. Adjusting the diet also helps, adding more hot energy foods. Think of red meat, lamb, ginger, black pepper and curry. Cooked food and hot drinks would also help. Warm foot baths and warming the abdomen with a hot water bottle for 15 minutes each evening are external means of warming the uterus.

Would you like to learn more about the concept of a cold uterus? Contact a natural medicine practitioner, such as an acupuncturist or Chinese medicine doctor (who specializes in women and fertility).

CHAPTER NINE

What you don't (and do) want to say to someone with fertility problems

Fertility problems. Although it is unfortunately still quite a taboo, we all know someone in our environment who does not want to have a child.

This can be uncomfortable for the environment, but extremely painful for the parents involved. Some advice can be completely wrong, but on the other hand, many women with fertility problems report that they often feel very alone in the process.

Fertility Problems

How do you best deal with this as an outsider? We give you a few clear do's & don'ts:

don't:

And big no—no:

The relativity.

"Oh, don't worry, it will come naturally." Or: "You are still so young!" Or also recognizable: "You are too busy with it, just let it go!" This kind of advice usually always goes down the wrong way with women. The point at which you can still be nonchalant about having children is long gone. Age also doesn't matter. Women have a wish, and no matter how old they are, it's very sad when it doesn't seem to work out .

Complaining about motherhood.

"My kids are so busy every day, take one of mine!" Or: "I really underestimated how heavy a second child would be." Sure, everyone can complain once in a while, but these are complaints that women with fertility problems cannot relate to. Pick your audience.

Share pregnancy news openly.

"Look, Meghan Markle is already pregnant 3 months after her wedding!" Or: "Wow, check out that friend's pregnancy announcement on Instagram!" We guarantee that this will not always go down well with women who are unable to conceive. Think about this. Pregnancy announcements, on the other hand, confront these women with the facts, which can make it difficult for them to be uninhibitedly happy.

Avoid news

However, what you should also not do: avoid news of a new pregnancy. In this way, the woman in question can feel very excluded again. So bring it in a slightly more subtle way. Feel this situation. So never bring pregnancy news in public. Give her time to process it. With some friendships this is via whatsapp or a card. In other cases, calling or visiting her home is more appropriate. For example, we know an example of two friends, one of whom had difficulty having a child. When the other turned out to be pregnant, she brought the news face—to—face, with a large bunch of flowers. A very thoughtful gesture!

Do or say nothing.

This may be the worst thing you can do once a friend shares her fertility issues with you. She probably mustered up some courage to bring this subject up for discussion. Silence is then extra painful. But what do you say?

Tips below.

dos

Then what?

Leave her in charge.

If your friend brings up her fertility issues, leave her in the lead on what she does and doesn't want to share. Also be honest about the fact that you don't want to hurt her feelings and that she certainly doesn't have to answer questions you ask her if she doesn't want to. However, do ask those questions. This way your girlfriend feels taken seriously. You can also ask her if she appreciates it if you occasionally raise the subject with her. Some women like this and feel supported by it. Others want to be left alone more during the process and don't want to have to announce every month that "it didn't work out again."

Try to support her in tough decisions.

Whether your friend chooses fertility treatment or not, support her in this decision. Let her know and ask questions about the treatment and the period ahead. Ask regularly how she is feeling. You can keep well—intentioned advice such as: do you know how much IVF can cost and how hard it can be physically and mentally. Trust us: your girlfriend knows about this.

Distract group conversations from babies.

If your girlfriend has confided in you about her desire to have children, you can assume that she does not want you to share this with others. Nor will she share this with everyone for a long time. For example, often enough group conversations can arise in which uninhibited baby news and talk is shared. Help your girlfriend by subtly changing the topic of conversation.

Try to distract your girlfriend.

If your girlfriend has been trying to get pregnant for some time, you will notice that the time is ticking by too slowly. Especially the last weeks of the cycle, just before menstruation (or pregnancy!) can be nerve—wracking. Try to distract her with lunch, a movie, a shopping afternoon or dinner. This way you give her the feeling without using your words that her life without wanting children can also be very nice.

Can you feel your cervix to see if you are pregnant?

If you are trying to conceive, you will find that you are quite alert to changes in your body in the weeks following ovulation. Do you have sore breasts? More discharge than usual? Or a stomach cramp? It can be quite difficult to predict in advance whether you are pregnant or not.

Many women become very restless because of this, and actively look for signs. For example, can you feel your cervix to see if you are pregnant? We figured it out.

CHAPTER TEN

How you feel your cervix

Feeling the position of your cervix can sometimes be a difficult job. It is also important that you do it more often, to really feel a difference. Ideally, do it the same way and at the same time. Ways to feel your cervix well are by squatting, or with one leg on the edge of the toilet or bath. Insert one or two fingers and gently feel the area,

Your cervix during your cycle

Just as your body changes constantly during your menstrual cycle under the influence of hormones, so does your cervix.

It is well known that if you want to get pregnant, the

position of your cervix can tell you a lot about where you are in your cycle.

After your period you will notice that your cervix is still fairly high and slightly open. As the bleeding completely passes, you will notice that your cervix sags, becoming hard and pointed. This is then completely closed. Have you ever given birth? Then it sometimes happens that your cervix no longer closes completely, but that a line can always be felt. If you have not given birth before, the cervix will feel completely closed.

As you move closer to ovulation, you will notice that you sit higher and higher. Sometimes so far that you can't quite reach it with your finger. You feel that the cervix is more open, and around it you feel more stretchy mucus. The cervix also feels much softer than normal. This means that you are fertile, and you will ovulate within a few days.

After ovulation you will notice that your cervix closes again, and will feel hard and pointed again. It will also drop again.

Your cervix during pregnancy

Many women who want to have children cannot resist feeling the cervix when ovulation has taken place. However, it is difficult to determine whether you are pregnant based on the position of your cervix. There is no specific maxim about what exactly the position should be when you are pregnant. Pregnant women's experiences vary widely.

For example, many women experience a high position, which feels fairly soft, while others feel a low position and a very hard cervix. Some feel that the cervix is completely closed, while others describe a 'swollen, soft feeling'.

So can you predict a pregnancy from the position of your uterus? Unfortunately, this has never been scientifically proven. The most reliable way to know if you are pregnant is still a pregnancy test.

You are pregnant! But what now? These are the first things you can do

The pregnancy test is positive and you are jumping up and down, but is this a reaction of joy or worry? Where one swoons away with her love, the other panics. yet everyone who is just pregnant asks themselves the same question; what's next ?

The first appointment with the midwife is only between the eighth and tenth week of pregnancy and they will answer a lot of questions for you, but in the meantime you can already do a lot yourself. That is why we have prepared a list for you to help you on your way in the time before the first appointment with the midwife.

Health

As you can understand, your own health is now extra important. You are now not only taking care of yourself, but also of the growth of the little creature in your belly.

1. Check your insurance

If you have not yet done so, check with your insurance whether or not you will be reimbursed.

2. Midwife

Find a great midwife and schedule an intake interview. Keep in mind that these people will assist you throughout the pregnancy and delivery, so choose one that you feel comfortable with. You can always switch if you find out that it doesn't click. So don't feel any discomfort. After all, it's about your pregnancy!

3. Sports

Do you sport? Then keep doing this, but maybe pay a little attention with abdominal exercises. Haven't you done this yet? Then see if you can find a sport that you feel comfortable with. It is very good to keep moving. But, don't feel obligated either. Your baby will also come out without you exercising.

Take time for yourself

You are often a lot more tired than before and that is for a reason. Your body uses all the energy to make the little one feel good, so give in to the fatigue and take a rest.

5. Medicines

Do you take medication? Check with your doctor or doctor whether this is safe in combination with your pregnancy.

6. Litter Box

Do you have a cat at home? Then it is better to leave the cleaning of the litter box to your sweetheart from now on (not such a problem in itself of course!). This is related to the risk of Toxoplasmosis.

7. Traveling

Now's the time! Have you already planned a trip? Or do you now see your chance to travel the world alone or with your partner? Above all, do it. But be aware that as a pregnant woman you are more vulnerable and more susceptible to diseases. In addition, Zika is still present in many places, so make sure you are well informed before you travel.

Wash

To prevent infectious diseases, it is important that you

wash your hands well. For example, after preparing food, after going to the toilet or after changing a diaper. In addition, it is also better to wash all fresh products extra well during your pregnancy. Think of fruits and vegetables.

9. Gardening

Do you enjoy rooting in your garden with your hands? During your pregnancy, make sure that you always use garden gloves and wash your hands well afterwards. This again in connection with the risk of Toxoplasmosis and Listeria.

Nutrition and early pregnancy

Nutrition, an important topic during your pregnancy.

1. Vitamins

If you haven't started this yet, start taking folic acid and vitamin D now.

2. Conscious eating

Start eating more mindfully. Rather leave the ready meals for a while and cook (or have them cooked for you) with fresh ingredients.

3. Be careful with certain foods

Be careful with foods that you should not eat during pregnancy. Such as raw meat and raw fish.

4. Fiber

Eat lots of fiber. The bowel movement is a point of attention during your pregnancy and can cause a lot of trouble.

5. Alcohol and smoking

Quit alcohol and smoking. And drugs!

Just pregnant and your relationship

Your relationship has brought you to the point where you are now pregnant, but now that you are pregnant a lot is about to change.

1. Sex

Don't stop having sex! It will not harm the pregnancy or your little one.

2. Daydreaming

Dream away together about baby names, the design of the room, parenting styles, and so on.

3. Going out

Go out together a lot. There is a good chance that you will avoid this a lot less later in the pregnancy, when the back pain and other ailments get the upper hand.

4. Pregnancy course with your partner

Look for fun pregnancy classes that you can do together. These may be in high demand in your area and fill up quickly

beauty

1. Lubricate your belly

Look for a nice oil or cream that you can rub your belly with. Even if you don't have a tummy yet, you can't start early enough to take care of the skin and prepare it for the huge stretch that awaits it.

2. Hairdresser

Keep going to the hairdresser, but get good advice when

you want to color your hair. Some types of hair dye seem to be less good during your pregnancy.

Pregnancy Memories

1. Belly Photos

Take pictures of your abdomen weekly. You never know when it will start to grow, so if you start right away, you'll at least get the transformation.

2. Pregnancy Diary

Keep a pregnancy diary. There are all kinds of designed booklets where you can answer a number of questions per week, but you can of course also keep something in a notebook yourself. There is so much going on in the early pregnancy that you often forget most of it quickly. And how nice is it to compare the experiences later in a second pregnancy?

Just pregnant at work

1. Telling at work

You don't have to tell them straight away at work when

you're just pregnant. Officially, you don't have to tell us until three weeks before the start of your leave, but it is of course advisable to do this earlier. To be on the safe side, it is useful to take the 12—week limit into account. Then the greatest chance of miscarriage is over.

2. Who to tell

Whether you tell your own manager or the HR manager first is completely up to you. It mainly depends on your relationship with your supervisor. If you are afraid of a less enthusiastic response, you can already obtain information from the HR department about your rights and obligations with regard to the pregnancy and your leave. One thing is certain; tell your supervisor before you announce it to all your colleagues.

CHAPTER ELEVEN

These are the pros and cons of fertility treatments abroad

An infertility problem comes with a lot of grief and frustration. Although more and more treatments are available in the Netherlands over the years, couples are increasingly opting for fertility treatments abroad.

What are the pros and cons of fertility treatments abroad? Why are more and more couples opting for cross—border treatment? We list the pros and cons.

The benefits of fertility treatment abroad

The waiting times for certain treatments are sometimes shorter abroad. This mainly relates to the waiting time for donor sperm or eggs.

Some treatments are possible abroad, but not in the

Netherlands. An example of this is the use of an anonymous sperm donor.

Abroad, more diagnostic research is often done to find out why a woman does not become pregnant than in the Netherlands.

In general, the Netherlands is more directing the fertility process. This means that doctors in the Netherlands sometimes choose to stop treatment if they consider the chance of pregnancy too small. Abroad, the patient's autonomy is often more central. This means that as long as the patient wants, treatment is possible for longer.

Different or more techniques are used to bring about a pregnancy than in the Netherlands. Think of 'assisted hatching', or 'scratching.' You can read more about the different treatments that are offered abroad here.

To increase the chances of a pregnancy, more embryos are often transferred abroad during IVF or ICSI treatment than in the Netherlands.

The disadvantages of fertility treatment abroad

The process of treatment abroad is more complicated. As a prospective parent, you would do well to compare different clinics and to contact these authorities to have all your questions answered. There may be a language barrier if you choose a foreign clinic.

It is not always clear whether treatment abroad is reimbursed. If you, as a prospective parent, do not investigate this properly, you may be surprised with very high costs.

Treatment abroad can be very intensive due to the travel time. For some treatments it may be necessary to stay there for several weeks in a row.

Abroad, other or more treatments are often offered than in the Netherlands, but do these really have added value for your specific situation?

Treatments abroad are even more often in an experimental phase. This is often the reason why they are not yet offered in the Netherlands. At first glance, these treatments may lead to better results, but the long—term effects are not always known.

Foreign clinics often continue with treatments longer than in the Netherlands. This can be an advantage, but it can also lead to false hopes.

Abroad, more than 1 embryo is often replaced during an IVF or ICSI treatment. This means a higher chance of a pregnancy, but a multiple pregnancy can also lead to more complications during the pregnancy and may pose a higher risk to your unborn babies.

Whether you ultimately opt for treatment abroad or not is a choice that you or your partner have to make. Many prospective parents move abroad because they want to feel that they have tried all options.

Discuss the advantages and disadvantages with each other, seek advice from your own doctor in the Netherlands and contact possible foreign clinics. Make sure you make your choice as informed as possible.

Thank You

Thank you for allowing me to be part of your fertility journey. I know this road can be filled with ups and downs, but I hope this book has helped bring you clarity, confidence, and a sense of empowerment.

Please remember: you are stronger than you think, and your body is capable of amazing things. Continue nourishing yourself with patience, care, and the right foods, and trust that you are doing something truly powerful for your health and future family.

If you found this guide helpful, I would be incredibly grateful if you left an honest review on Amazon —your feedback not only helps me, but also helps other women and couples who are looking for guidance and hope.

Wishing you all the best on your journey to parenthood! With love and encouragement,

Clare Dominic

xcix

FERTILITY DIET, THE INFERTILITY KILLER